THE FOUNDATION
Nutrition & Health
HANDBOOK

Dr Mabel Blades

PhD, RD, MBA, BSc, MPhil, DMS, FRSH, FIFST

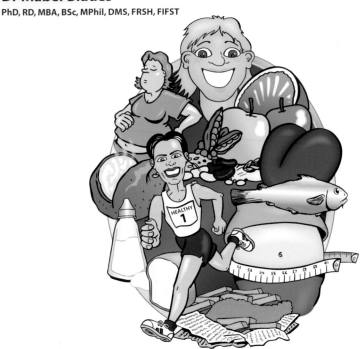

First published 2006

"Vue Pointe", Spinney Hill, Sprotbrough, Doncaster, South Yorkshire, DN5 7LY, U.K.
Tel: +44 0845 2260350 Fax: +44 0845 2260360
E-mail: info@highfield.co.uk
ISBN 1-904544-51-7

Printed by Trafford Press Tel: 01302 367509

www.highfield.co.uk

www.foodsafetytrainers.co.uk

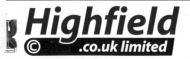

Improving Your Health

CONTENTS

Brian

Anjana

Julie

Lindsey

Good health is of supreme importance to us all.

Food, nutrition and diet ▼

What we eat is vital to our health and well-being as well as to how we look, feel and function. If we do not feel good then it means that we are not getting the most out of life and not doing all those things we really want to do.

Also it is essential that we actually enjoy our food and feel satisfied by it and are not just feeling constantly hungry and not really enjoying the food we eat.

Eight guidelines for a healthy diet ▼

The Food Standards Agency (FSA) adopted 'Eight Guidelines for a Healthy Diet' which have recently been updated as '8 tips for eating well':

1. Base your meals on starchy foods.
2. Eat lots of fruit and vegetables.
3. Eat more fish.
4. Cut down on saturated fat and sugar.
5. Try to eat less salt – no more than 6g a day.
6. Get active and try to be a healthy weight.
7. Drink plenty of water.
8. Don't skip breakfast.

QUESTION

What people would the knowledge of nutrition be helpful for?

ANSWER

- **HEALTH CARE STAFF,** e.g. nurses, carers, ward hostesses, catering managers, dietetic assistants
- **CARE HOMES,** e.g. carers, cooks
- **CATERERS OF ALL TYPES,** e.g. hospital caterers, caterers in care homes, school meals staff, prison service caterers
- **STAFF IN THE RETAIL INDUSTRY,** e.g. supermarkets
- **HOSPITALITY INDUSTRY,** e.g. restaurants
- **LEISURE INDUSTRY,** e.g. fitness instructors, slimming group leaders
- **PUBLIC RELATIONS & ADVERTISING INDUSTRY,** e.g. copywriters dealing with food and diet
- **EDUCATION,** e.g. catering managers, catering supervisors, teachers

Although the word diet has become synonymous with a slimming diet in the context of the study of nutrition, it means the normal foods and beverages consumed each day.

Healthy eating and a healthy diet ▼

It is generally recognised that there are no unhealthy foods, only unbalanced and therefore unhealthy diets. So it is the amount of different foods that people eat that can cause problems.

There is nothing wrong with the occasional bar of chocolate or fried breakfast but when fried foods and chocolate are taken frequently the diet can become high in fat.

The balance of good health ▼

The *Balance of Good Health* is a pictorial illustration of a well-balanced and healthy diet. It shows the 5 main food groups and the proportions of each of the foods that are recommended to be eaten as part of a healthy diet.

These food groups include:

- fruit and vegetables;
- bread, other cereals and potatoes;
- milk and dairy foods;
- meat, fish and alternatives; and
- foods containing fat and foods and drinks containing sugar.

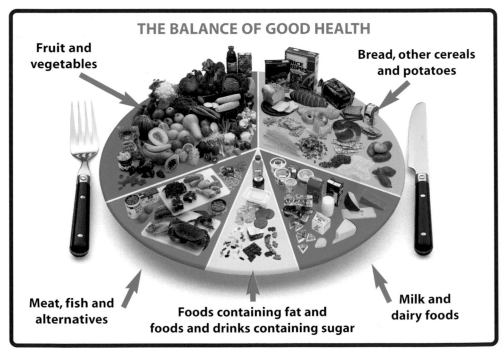

THE BALANCE OF GOOD HEALTH

Fruit and vegetables

Bread, other cereals and potatoes

Meat, fish and alternatives

Foods containing fat and foods and drinks containing sugar

Milk and dairy foods

As can be seen from the illustration of the *Balance of Good Health* the largest proportions of food that should be eaten as part of a healthy diet are fruit and vegetables and bread, other cereals and potatoes.

The *Balance of Good Health* focuses on food not nutrients but in general the 5 food groups contain the following nutrients:

- fruit and vegetables - do provide vitamins, minerals, some dietary fibre or non-starch polysaccharide (NSP) and carbohydrate;
- bread, other cereals and potatoes - do provide carbohydrate of a starchy type, some dietary fibre or non-starch polysaccharides (NSP) especially if these are unrefined foods, vitamins, minerals and protein;
- milk and dairy foods - do provide protein and vitamins and minerals particularly calcium. They also provide a source of fat if they are full fat types;
- meat, fish and alternatives - do provide protein and minerals especially iron as well as vitamins; and
- foods containing fat and foods containing sugar - do provide fat, particularly saturated fats and also sugars.

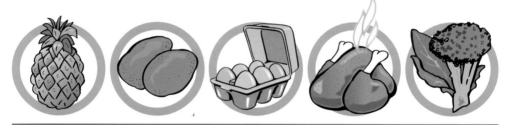

QUESTION

What do you eat?
List the fruit and vegetables you have eaten in the last week.
List the starchy carbohydrates that you have eaten in the last week.
List the milk and dairy foods that you have eaten in the last week.
List the meat, fish and alternatives that you have eaten in the last week.
List the fats and sugary foods that you have eaten in the last week.
Which of the foods do you eat in the biggest amounts?
Is it the fruits and vegetables or the fats and sugars?

ANSWER

Ideally you should have 5 portions of fruit and vegetables each day. Plenty of starchy carbohydrates. Some milk and dairy foods (preferably low fat varieties, meat, fish and alternatives and not too many foods containing fat and sugar).

Health problems related to a poor diet ▼

Unfortunately the average diet eaten in this country is not reflective of that illustrated in the *Balance of Good Health*. Many people eat too much fat, especially too much saturated fat, too little fruit and vegetables and not enough bread, other cereals and potatoes and too much sugar, salt and alcohol.

There are major links between diet and health problems such as obesity, coronary heart disease, high blood pressure, strokes and certain cancers.

1. Obesity ▼

Usually due to too many calories from food and too little activity. Approximately 50% of the adult population are overweight or obese.

High calorie foods such as fatty foods, excess alcohol and an inactive lifestyle are particularly to blame.

2. Coronary heart disease ▼

This is linked with:
- too much saturated fat in the diet;
- too few antioxidant vitamins from such foods as fruit and vegetables;
- being obese;
- inactivity;
- smoking;
- family history; and
- males.

3. High blood pressure and strokes ▼

This is an increasing problem among adults and contributes to serious problems such as strokes. It is linked with:
- obesity; and
- too much salt from convenience foods, salty snacks and adding salt at the table to foods.

4. Certain cancers ▼

Various cancers are found in different parts of the body. Some are strongly linked with diet. Fruit and vegetables and the antioxidants they contain are considered to have a preventative effect for cancer developing.

Cancers are also related to smoking, obesity and too much fat in the diet.

Bowel cancer is related to too little fibre in the diet.

QUESTION

Think of all the people you know who have a problem with diseases related to a poor diet. You will realise how common it is.

ANSWER

People with obesity, coronary heart disease, bowel cancer, anaemias, dental disease.

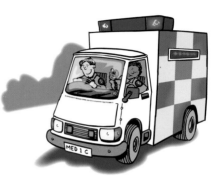

Vitamin C, beta-carotene, vitamin E and the mineral selenium all act as antioxidants. In addition, other antioxidants are found in plants and thus fruit and vegetables; for example, the antioxidant lycopene is found in tomatoes.

Antioxidants help to prevent diseases such as cancers and heart disease starting by mopping up harmful substances produced in the body.

QUESTION

Fruit and vegetables are a major source of antioxidants and fibre. Everyone is encouraged to have at least 5 portions per day. This is 400g in weight.
Look at your own diet and count up the number of portions of fruit and vegetables you eat each day.

ANSWER

If you are not having 5 portions try to have more by including fruit juice, extra fruit on cereal, in puddings and as snacks, as well as vegetables with meals.

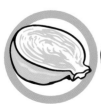
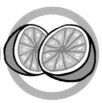
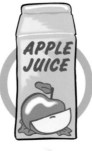
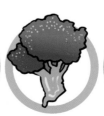

Fluid ▼

Fluid is needed for survival and without adequate fluid we can only survive a few days at most.

About 2 litres of fluid (3 pints) 6-8 cups or glasses of fluid is needed each day.

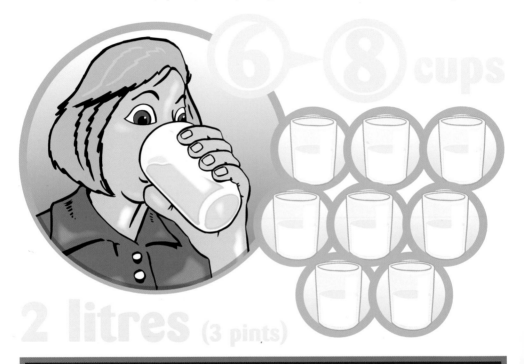

QUESTION

Add up the number of cups and glasses of liquid you take each day.

ANSWER

It should be 6-8 cups, mugs or glasses.

NOTE: Alcohol does not count as it causes the body to lose fluids via the kidneys. Beverages like teas, coffees, colas and chocolate drinks all contain caffeine which acts as a diuretic. This means it causes the kidneys to produce more urine and hence the body retains less fluid. The best fluid to rehydrate the body is water.

Nutrients ▼

There are 5 main groups of nutrients ▼

- Protein
- Fat
- Carbohydrate
- Vitamins
- Minerals

Energy is provided by protein, fat and carbohydrate. Fat provides 9 kcal per g, protein 4 kcal per g, with carbohydrate, 3.75 kcal per g. Alcohol is not a necessary part of the diet but it also provides energy of 7 kcal per g.

Vitamins and minerals are both vital for life but do not provide energy.

Foods are normally mixtures of a number of nutrients. Therefore a variety of different foods is required as part of a balanced diet. No one food is able to sustain adult life. Babies are able to thrive on breast milk for the first few months of life only.

Micronutrients are the nutrients which are required in small amounts, these include vitamins and minerals.

Trace elements or trace minerals are those minerals which are needed in minute amounts.

> ### MAIN MINERALS REQUIRED
> - **Calcium**
> - **Phosphorus**
> - **Sodium**
> - **Potassium**
> - **Iron**
> - **Zinc**
> - **Selenium***
> - **Iodine***
> - **Fluoride***
>
> * Trace elements or trace minerals

Units of measurements ▼

As with many other subjects, measurements are required and nutrition has a number of standard ways of measuring items.

Weights of foods and also of nutrients are measured in kilograms, grams, milligrams and micrograms.

Energy is measured in calories and joules. This measurement of energy can be either the energy obtained from macronutrients such as protein, fat, carbohydrate or alcohol or the energy expended in activities such as walking.

Energy derived from foods is normally quoted as kilocalories (kcal) per 100g of food. The energy for activities is normally quoted on food labels for the duration of time of the activity.

If we take in too much energy (calories) from food, we store up that extra energy as body fat. This fat is deposited around vital organs and below the skin on the abdomen, thighs, legs and other parts of the body.

Having excessive amounts of fat deposited on the body is called obesity. This has a number of health risks associated with it.

QUESTION

Can you think of health risks associated with obesity?

ANSWER

- Heart disease
- Hypertension
- Joint problems
- Breathlessness
- Type 2 diabetes
- Strokes
- Varicose veins
- Accidents
- Certain cancers
- Poor recovery from surgery
- Psychological problems
- Social problems

Dietary Reference Values for food energy and nutrients for the UK ▼

This report is a key document as it gives standards upon which to base the nutritional content of diets for groups such as those in schools and also for individuals. The report was produced by the Panel on Dietary Reference Values of the Committee of the Medical Aspects of Food Policy, which is often referred to as COMA, in 1991.

It contains a range of figures giving the various amounts of nutrients needed for a healthy diet.

Energy ▼

The basic requirements of the body are often known as physiological requirements. This means the nutrients that we need to keep us alive.

To live we need energy for body activities. This energy is derived from foods.

DIETARY REFERENCE VALUES FOR FOOD ENERGY AND NUTRIENTS FOR THE UNITED KINGDOM (1991) COMA

- **DRV** **Dietary Reference Values includes EAR & RNI**
- **EAR** **Estimated Average Requirement**
- **RNI** **Reference Nutrient Intake**

The figures in the report on Dietary Reference Values provide information which has been derived from examination of numerous reports on nutrition on the amounts of energy and nutrients required by different age groups of the population and for males and females. The report also makes recommendations as to the proportions of energy which should be derived from different macronutrients like carbohydrates and fats.

Proportions of energy, which should be derived from different nutrients ▼

A greater proportion of our energy derived from food should be obtained from starchy carbohydrates such as bread, potatoes, rice, pasta and breakfast cereals. In fact 45-50% of calories in the diet should be obtained from carbohydrates.

As can be seen, the group with the highest requirements for energy are males aged 15 to 18 years as they normally are very active and are also growing.

It must however be remembered that these figures are an average and do not take into account individual variations. As an average figure it means that half of a population will need more than the figure given and half will need less.

Reference Nutrient Intakes (RNI) ▼

The RNI is the term used to indicate the amount of protein, vitamins and minerals required for 97% of the population.

ENERGY REQUIREMENTS

Age	Males kcal/day	Females kcal/day
0-3 months	545	515
4-6 months	690	645
7-9 months	825	765
10-12 months	920	865
1-3 years	1230	1165
4-6 years	1715	1545
7-10 years	1970	1740
11-14 years	2220	1845
15-18 years	2755	2110
19-50 years	2550	1940
51-59 years	2550	1900
60-64 years	2380	1900
65-74 years	2330	1900
75+ years	2100	1810

Pregnancy last 13 weeks extra 200 kcal per day.
Breast-feeding extra 450-570 kcal per day.

Metabolism ▼

The body is a complex living structure composed of billions of individual cells. The cells themselves consist of proteins and other nutrients bound together in certain ways that gives each cell its own special function.

Cells are grouped together into tissues and organs which perform specific functions; for example, the skin is the largest tissue in the body, while the heart is the organ responsible for the circulation of blood.

Within the body, chemical reactions are occurring all the time in cells to enable them to carry out the processes of growth and repair needed for life. This complex collection of chemical reactions is called metabolism.

Energy is required for metabolism to occur. The energy is derived from foods such as carbohydrates, proteins and fats. Alcohol also provides energy.

Basal Metabolic Rate (BMR) ▼

Energy is required for all of the metabolic actions to occur in the body. These processes include the basic ones required to keep us alive and include:

- breathing;
- heartbeat;
- maintenance of body temperature;
- brain activities; and
- secretion of enzymes.

These activities are occurring all the time and as we are not aware of them they are referred to as involuntary activities. They all require energy and the amount of energy required is called the Basal Metabolic Rate, which is often abbreviated as the BMR.

Energy requirements ▼

Everyone needs energy from food to live. Energy is required for all of the vital functions of the body such as maintenance of the body temperature, breathing, digestion, blood circulation, hormone release and all of the other cellular activities that occur in the body.

Additionally we need energy for all the activities such as movements whether small ones such as reading or more vigorous ones such as jogging.

Energy is also needed for growth such as occurs in children and during pregnancy.

Energy is measured in both kilojoules and megajoules abbreviated as kJ and MJ respectively. Also energy is measured in kilocalories, abbreviated as kcal. The latter term is usually referred to as 'calories' and is familiar to anyone who has tried to control their calorie intake in an effort to lose weight.

The simple way of converting energy in kilocalories to kilojoules (to give a good approximation) is to multiply by 4.2. Thus a food such as a digestive biscuit, which contains 70 kilocalories would provide about 294 kilojoules.

Energy is obtained from foods and is needed for the maintenance of life. This requirement includes the energy needed for basic metabolic activities plus additional activities such as movements of the body, which require muscular activity. Such activities include reading, walking, running and driving.

Foods providing energy ▼

Protein, fat and carbohydrate all provide energy.

Protein provides 4 kilocalories of energy per gram and carbohydrate provides 3.75 kilocalories per gram and fat 9 kilocalories per gram.

As can be seen, fat provides a much more concentrated source of energy than protein or carbohydrate. This is why it forms body stores for energy.

Percentage energy from fat in the diet ▼

For a healthy diet we are recommended to limit the amount of fat, especially saturated fat, due to the links between fat and coronary heart disease. The recommended source of energy is from starchy carbohydrates such as bread, potatoes, pasta and rice. Carbohydrates should provide 45-50% of energy.

It is recommended that the maximum percentage of the total amount of energy provided by fat in the diet is a maximum of 35%. Protein should provide about 15% of energy if taken, while alcohol should provide no more than 5% of energy.

Proteins, fats and carbohydrates ▼

Proteins ▼

Humans need a regular supply of protein in their diet. The main sources of proteins are meats, offal, poultry, fish, eggs, cheese, milk and yoghurts. For vegetarians and vegans, nuts and pulses such as peas, beans and lentils all provide protein. Potatoes, rice, fruit and green vegetables are all shown to contain relatively low levels of protein.

The main sources of proteins are:
- meats;
- offal;
- poultry;
- fish;
- eggs;
- cheese;
- milk; and
- yoghurts.

For vegetarians and vegans, nuts and pulses such as:
- peas;
- beans; and
- lentils all provide protein.

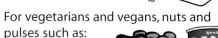

> ## QUESTION
>
> *Where are proteins found in the human body?*
>
> ### ANSWER
>
> - About 43% of body proteins are found in the muscle tissues
> - 21% in the skin
> - 19% in the blood
> - 5% in the liver
> - Brain
> - Kidneys
> - Hair
> - Nails
> - Other vital organs
> - Key components of hormones
> - Enzymes such as digestive enzymes
> - Part of the immune system (the immune system is responsible for helping the body to fight off infections and illnesses) is made up of proteins

The following table shows the percentage of protein in various foods:

FOOD	PERCENTAGE OF PROTEIN
Cod frozen raw	16.7%
Salmon raw	20.2%
Lamb, average extra trimmed lean, raw	20.0%
Pork, average, trimmed lean raw	21.8%
Beef, average, extra trimmed lean, raw	21.6
Chicken, meat, average raw	23.3
Cashew nuts	17.7%
Lentils, red, dried, raw, uncooked	23.8%
Eggs raw	12.5%
Cheese cheddar, average	25.5%
Semi-skimmed milk, pasteurized, average	3.3%
Dried skimmed milk	36.1%
White rice raw, uncooked	6.5%
White bread	8.4%
Macaroni raw, uncooked	12.0%
Cauliflower raw	3.6%
New potatoes average raw	1.7%
Apples eating raw	0.4%

Tissue proteins of the body are continually being broken down and reformed. Therefore humans need a regular supply of protein in their diet.

The Reference Nutrient Intake for protein is 55.5g per day in adult males aged 19-50 years and 55.3g in those males over 50 years of age. The reference nutrient intake for protein is 45.0g per day in adult females aged 19-50 years and 46.5g in those females over 50 years of age. During pregnancy an extra 6.0g of protein per day is required. In the first four months of breast-feeding this requirement increases to 11g of protein per day.

In general this recommendation is based on a figure of 0.75g/protein per kg/body weight per day.

During periods of injury or infection more protein may be needed.

Amino acids ▼

Proteins are made up of chains of amino acids. Some of these amino acids are called indispensable or essential amino acids as they cannot be made in the body but must be supplied by the diet. There are 8 such amino acids in adults and 9 in children.

Foods containing all of the essential amino acids are ones in foods such as meat, offal, fish, milk, eggs and cheese.

Vegetable foods such as pulses (peas, beans and lentils) may have a limited content of one of the essential amino acids and therefore this needs to be supplied by other foods in the diet.

Eight essential amino acids

Eight essential amino acids for adults:

- Isoleucine
- Phenylalanine
- Leucine
- Threonine
- Lysine
- Tryptophan
- Methionine
- Valine

Histidine is indispensable for infants because of their rapid growth rate

Sources of protein ▼

The major sources of protein in the diet are meat, eggs, fish, cheese and pulses.

Fats ▼

All fats provide 9 kcal per gram and are thus equal as regards a source of energy. Too much energy in the diet can contribute to weight gain as already described. We should take no more than 35% of the energy from fat in the diet.

Saturated fats are derived from animal sources such as full cream milks, full fat cheese, lard, butter, the fat found on meat and other fatty foods. This is the type of fat associated with coronary heart disease. Coconut and palm oils also contain saturated fat.

Polyunsaturated fats are those derived from plant oils such as soya, corn and soya oils. These oils are felt to be beneficial but still provide a source of calories.

Monounsaturated fats are found in olive oil and rapeseed oil. Such fats are felt to be beneficial to the heart.

Typical fatty acid composition of some foods

FOOD	g/100g food	Fatty acids (% of fat by weight)		
		Saturated	Monounsaturated	Polyunsaturated
Butter	82.2	72	25	3
Margarine, soft	80.0	35	47	18
Margarine, *polyunsaturated*	68.5	25	23	52
Rapeseed oil	99.9	7	62	31
Sunflower oil	99.9	13	21	66
Milk, whole cows'	4.0	71	26	3
Eggs	11.2	35	47	18
Cheese, Cheddar	32.7	71	26	3
Beef, mince	15.7	51	47	2
Pork, chops	15.7	38	44	18
Biscuits, choc chip	22.9	49	39	12
Potato crisps	11.0	68	30	2
Peanuts	46.0	20	50	30

Essential fatty acids ▼

Certain polyunsaturated fatty acids are called essential as they cannot be made by the body and therefore must be provided by the diet.

They are involved in making cell membranes in the body.

Omega 3 and Omega 6 fatty acids ▼

Omega 3 fatty acids are particularly helpful in preventing coronary heart disease. Sources of omega 3 fatty acids are fish oils, particularly those from oily fish. Oily fish are mackerel, fresh tuna (not canned), trout, salmon, pilchards and sardines.

Omega 6 fatty acids can also prevent coronary heart disease. Sources of omega 6 fatty acids are sunflower oil, corn oil and soya oils.

Cholesterol ▼

Cholesterol is a sticky wax-like substance and is essential to life and is:

- a component of cell walls;
- needed for the synthesis of bile salts necessary for fat digestion;
- required for the production of steroid hormones; and
- manufacturer of vitamin D in the body.

Cholesterol circulates in the blood and a measurement of it indicates a risk of coronary heart disease. There are two types of cholesterol:
- low density lipoprotein (LDL), the bad type of cholesterol; and
- high density lipoprotein cholesterol (HDL) which is the good type of cholesterol.

A high proportion of saturated fat in the diet predisposes the production of bad cholesterol.

Cholesterol is found in relatively few foods. Food sources of cholesterol are egg yolks, liver and shellfish.

A certain amount of fat is needed in the diet to provide the essential fatty acids, which are vital in the production of cell membranes in the body.

The fat-soluble vitamins A,D,E and K are found alongside fats in the diet.

Fat is a source of energy in the diet and as they provide 9 kcal per g fats are the most concentrated form of energy in the diet (protein provides 4 kcal per g and carbohydrate 3.75 kcal per g).

If we take in too much energy from food in our diet the body stores this up as fat in adipose tissue. Adipose tissue is found below the skin and excessive quantities can be deposited in the abdominal area. The excessive deposition of body fat is termed obesity.

We are encouraged to reduce the level of fat in our diet.

QUESTION

What fats are in the diet and where they are found?

ANSWER

Butter	Low fat spreads, these	Cheese *(even	Pastry, cakes & biscuits
Lard & oil	contain 25-70% fat	low fat cheddar	Cheese spread
Fat on meat	Polyunsaturated	cheese contains	Ice cream
Margarine	spread	approximately	Fried foods
Suet	Nuts & seeds	17% fat)*	Croquettes
Cream	Full fat milk (silver top)	Fatty meat	Samosas
Oily fish	Egg yolk	Sauces	Crisps & chips *(deep fried)*

QUESTION

What foods contain low levels of fat?

ANSWER

- All types of fruit and vegetables with the exception of olives and avocados
- Bread, potatoes, pasta, rice, breakfast cereals
- Lean red meat – pork, beef and lamb
- Poultry with no skin
- Rabbit and game
- Skimmed milk
- Cottage cheese
- Low fat yoghurts

QUESTION

Which cooking methods do not add fat to food?

ANSWER

- Steaming
- Poaching
- Braising
- Casseroling
- Baking
- Simmering
- Grilling
- Boiling
- Barbecuing
- Stewing
- Dry frying without fat

Carbohydrates ▼

There are 2 main types of carbohydrate, sugary ones and starchy ones. Sugary ones include sugar, jams, soft sugary drinks, sweets, cakes, scones, sweet biscuits and desserts. Sugary carbohydrates have been strongly linked with dental decay.

Starchy carbohydrates include bread, potatoes, pasta, breakfast cereals, rice and cous cous.

Both types of carbohydrate provide the same amount of energy (3.75 kcal per g). The preferred source of energy for health is starchy carbohydrates and most of the energy in the diet should be derived from starchy carbohydrates.

Foods containing starches:

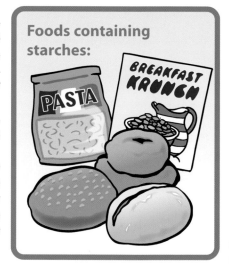

Foods containing sugar:

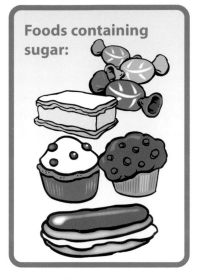

Therefore sugar is not required for energy.

Dietary fibre or non-starch polysaccharide (NSP) is also a form of carbohydrate. It does not provide energy as the body cannot break it down.

Sugars ▼

Sugars consist of both monosaccharides (sometimes called simple or single sugars) and disaccharides.

1. Sucrose is commonly seen as table sugar and is a disaccharide.
2. Lactose is found in milk both that from animals and also in human breast milk, it is also a dissaccharide.
3. Glucose is a monosaccharide.

Starches (polysaccharides) ▼

'Poly' means many and starches are made up of many units of glucose joined together. During this process of digestion, starches are broken down to their component glucose units.

Glycogen ▼

This is formed by the body in humans and animals from glucose. It is a form of polysaccharide, which is stored in small amounts in the liver and muscles to provide a temporary store of glucose for energy.

Dietary fibre or non-starch polysaccharide (NSP) ▼

We are all encouraged to take plenty of dietary fibre or non-starch polysaccharide (NSP) as it is correctly called. Dietary fibre used to be called roughage. This has a protective effect on the bowel and helps to prevent constipation, diverticular disease,

DIETARY FIBRE
(NON-STARCH POLYSACCHARIDE)

- **2 types**
- **Soluble fibre**
  oats, lentils, peas, dried beans, fruit and vegetables
- **Insoluble fibre**
  wholemeal bread, brown pasta, bran-based cereals e.g. branflakes

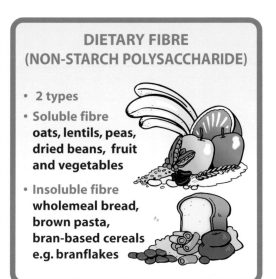

haemorrhoids and bowel cancer. We are advised to take about 18g of dietary fibre each day but on average we only take 12g.

There are 2 types of dietary fibre or NSP: Soluble fibre which has a beneficial effect on blood cholesterol and blood sugar levels. Insoluble fibre is helpful for bowel health. A number of people have problems such as diabetes with the associated raised blood sugar levels while others have heart diseases and raised cholesterol levels. Soluble fibre is helpful for them. Soluble fibre is found in all types of fruit and vegetables. Insoluble fibre is found in wholewheat products such as wholemeal bread.

Intrinsic and extrinsic sugars ▼

Intrinsic sugars are those contained in the structure of foods such as in fruits. Extrinsic sugars are those added in manufacturing foods such as in cakes.

Carbohydrate requirements ▼

At least half of the energy in our diets should come from carbohydrate, and mostly from starch. Thus at least 50% of the energy should be derived from carbohydrate.

Sources of carbohydrate ▼

Different foods contain different amounts of carbohydrate.

Sugars are naturally found in milk, honey and fruit but are also added to many prepared foods (e.g. biscuits, puddings, sweets and soft drinks).

Sources of starch include breakfast cereals and cereal foods (e.g. wheat, rice, maize, cassava, oats, rye, barley) roots and tubers (e.g. yams, potatoes, root vegetables), pulses (peas, beans and lentils) and some fruit.

QUESTION

What sources of sugar, starches and dietary fibre are there?

ANSWER

- Sugar - sweets, chocolate, cakes, pastries.
- Starches - bread, potatoes, pasta.

Dietary fibre in wholemeal bread, brown pasta, brown rice, wholegrain breakfast cereals, fruit, vegetables and dried fruit.

Vitamins and minerals ▼

Vitamins and minerals are essential but only needed in small amounts.

Vitamins ▼

Vitamins are essential to life: the name 'vitamin' is partly derived from the same root as the word 'vital'.

They are only needed in small amounts and are required for various metabolic functions in the body.

There are 2 major types of vitamins: fat soluble and water soluble vitamins.

Fat soluble vitamins are able to be stored in the liver and therefore do not require to be taken in the diet every day. Fat soluble vitamins are vitamin A, D, E and K.

Water soluble vitamins cannot be stored by the body and need to be taken regularly as part of the diet. These vitamins include the B vitamin group and vitamin C.

Water soluble vitamins

Vitamin C
Found in:
- **Citrus fruit, potatoes, vegetables, fruit and fruit juices.**

B vitamins
Found in:
- **Meat, wholegrain breakfast cereals, bread and rice.**

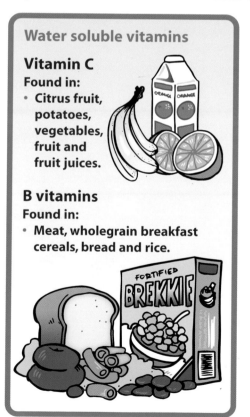

Fat soluble vitamins

Vitamin A
Found in:
- **Oily fish, margarine, eggs and liver.**

Vitamin D
Found in:
- **Oily fish, margarine, eggs and liver.**

Vitamin E
Found in:
- **Nuts and seeds.**

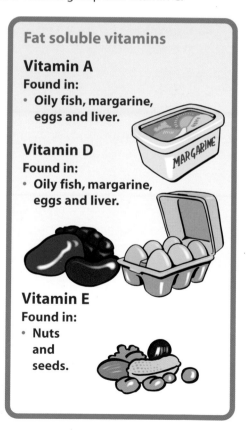

Vitamin C ▼

Vitamin C is needed for healthy skin and connective tissue (the tissue that binds cells together). It helps wound healing and the absorption of some forms of iron. It also acts as an antioxidant and this protects against coronary heart disease and cancers.

Vitamin C is found in fruit and vegetables especially citrus fruit.

B vitamins ▼

The B vitamins are needed for the release of energy from foods. Some B vitamins are needed for the formation of red blood cells.

The B vitamins are found particularly in wholegrain breads, cereals, meat, fish, yeast extracts and milk.

Vitamin A ▼

Vitamin A is needed for healthy eyes. It is also needed for tissue growth and repair. Vitamin A is found in butter, margarine, full fat milk, cream, cheese, eggs, liver ad oily fish. The body can make vitamin A from beta-carotene, the red/yellow substance found in carrots, apricots, tomatoes, mangoes and also green vegetables like broccoli.

Vitamin D ▼

Vitamin D is needed for the body to absorb calcium. It is made by the action of sunlight on the skin. Most people get enough this way unless they do not go out of doors. For those people who do not get it from sunlight a dietary source is required, such as full cream milk, margarine or oily fish.

Minerals ▼

The main minerals calcium, phosphorus, iron, sodium, potassium and zinc are all essential.

The minerals selenium, iodine and fluoride are all also essential but as they are only needed in tiny amounts, they are called trace minerals or elements.

Calcium and phosphorus ▼

Calcium combines with phosphorous to make calcium phosphate which is the hard material that gives hardness and strength to bones and teeth.

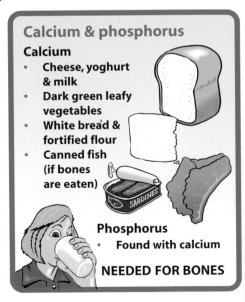

Calcium & phosphorus

Calcium
- **Cheese, yoghurt & milk**
- **Dark green leafy vegetables**
- **White bread & fortified flour**
- **Canned fish (if bones are eaten)**

Phosphorus
- **Found with calcium**

NEEDED FOR BONES

Calcium is required for blood clotting and correct functioning of muscles and nerves.

Calcium is found in good supply in milk, cheese, bread (added to white flour by law), bones of canned fish and hard water.

The absorption of calcium and phosphorous is controlled by vitamin D.

Calcium deficiency in children means that they have weak bones and rickets develop.

A lack of calcium can mean muscles and nerves do not function correctly which may result in cramps.

Iron ▼

Iron is needed in the form of haemoglobin, which carries oxygen to all cells of the body from the lungs.

There are 2 forms of dietary iron: haem iron and non-haem iron. The iron in red meat is in the haem form, and is well absorbed while the iron in cereals, vegetables and fruit are poorly absorbed. However if meat is eaten at the same meal as other foods then it actually enhances the absorption of iron from these other foods.

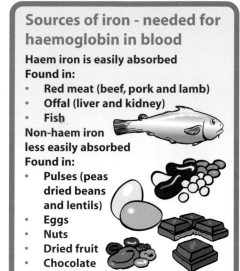

Sources of iron - needed for haemoglobin in blood

Haem iron is easily absorbed
Found in:
- **Red meat (beef, pork and lamb)**
- **Offal (liver and kidney)**
- **Fish**

Non-haem iron less easily absorbed
Found in:
- **Pulses (peas dried beans and lentils)**
- **Eggs**
- **Nuts**
- **Dried fruit**
- **Chocolate**

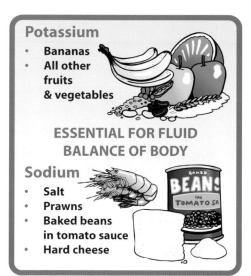

Potassium
- **Bananas**
- **All other fruits & vegetables**

ESSENTIAL FOR FLUID BALANCE OF BODY

Sodium
- **Salt**
- **Prawns**
- **Baked beans in tomato sauce**
- **Hard cheese**

Vitamin C also helps the absorption of iron in the non-haem form.

A lack of dietary iron can contribute to iron deficiency anaemia.

Iron deficiency anaemia is one of the most common nutritional deficiencies and particularly affects infants between 6 and 12 months, teenagers especially girls, women of menstruating age and elderly people.

Potassium and sodium ▼

Sodium is called an electrolyte and together with potassium it helps to maintain the fluid balance in the body.

Sodium is also required for nerve and muscle impulses. Most sodium is found in the fluid outside the cells.

Sodium is a major component of table salt, which is correctly called sodium chloride. There is approximately 1 gram of sodium in each 2.5 grams of sodium chloride. Sodium chloride is used extensively in cooking to bring out the flavour of foods and is also added to food at the table. Snacks such as crisps, savoury biscuits are popular and contribute to the sodium intake. Canned foods also contain increased levels of salt compared with fresh or frozen foods.

Other minerals ▼

Selenium (trace element) ▼

Selenium is an important antioxidant. Therefore like other antioxidants it has a protective effect against heart disease.

Selenium is found naturally in red meat. Fish and cereals contain selenium. Red meat is a good source of selenium. Brazil nuts are a rich source of selenium.

Zinc ▼

Zinc is a vital component in the functioning of the immune system of the body, which helps to fight diseases and infections. Zinc is also needed for the healing of wounds and the development of sexual maturity, particularly in males.

The most reliable source of zinc in the diet is from meat. Zinc in meat is in a form which is easily absorbed.

Fluoride (trace element) ▼

Fluoride has been shown to be an important factor in the strengthening of teeth against decay. It is thought that it combines with the protective enamel coating of the teeth thus making them more resistant to attack by the acid produced by bacteria in the mouth. For this reason fluoride has been added to drinking water and toothpastes.

Fluoride is found naturally in tea, sea water fish and in some parts of the country in water supplies. Tea provides most of the fluoride in the diet in this country.

Iodine (trace element) ▼

Iodine is required to make the hormone thyroxine which is produced by the thyroid gland in the neck. Thyroxine along with other hormones helps to control the rate of metabolism in the body.

Iodine is widely distributed in foods but is found in good supply in seafoods, milk, green vegetables, especially spinach, fresh water (depending upon area) and iodised salt (added commercially).

A deficiency of iodine leads to a reduction in the amount of thyroxine produced by the thyroid gland. This swelling was commonly found in areas such as Switzerland and Derbyshire in the past.

Digestion and absorption ▼

Before we can obtain any nourishment or nutrients from our foods they need to be digested and absorbed.

Digestion is the process whereby the body breaks down the foods which are eaten in the digestive tract, into the small components which can then be absorbed.

The absorption of the vitamins and minerals, simple sugars like glucose, amino acids and fats mainly occurs in the small intestine.

Conditions affecting the digestive tract ▼

- IBS can be helped by people taking plenty of fibre, especially soluble fibre and fluid.
- Ulcers can be helped by regular meals with no hot spicy foods.
- Constipation can be helped by people taking plenty of fibre and fluid.
- Coeliac disease is an intolerance to gluten found in wheat, rye, and barley. It can be helped by avoiding foods such as bread which contains them.

DIGESTIVE TRACT

Digestive tract and small intestine

FOOD

Villi

Blood Vessels

Under a microscope the small intestine looks like this.

Food is absorbed into the blood system through the villi.

Mouth
Oesophagus
Liver
Stomach
Gall bladder
Pancreas
Large intestine
Small intestine
Anus

QUESTION

Can you think of any problems affecting the digestive tract?

ANSWER

Irritable bowel syndrome, ulcers, cancers, constipation, food poisoning, coeliac disease, ulcerative colitis, cystic fibrosis, gallstones, food allergies and intolerances.

Foods groups ▼

Fruits and vegetables ▼

These provide vitamins, e.g. vitamin C, carotenes, folates, some minerals and dietary fibre.

The fruit and vegetables can be fresh, frozen or canned. Fruit and vegetables contain a variety of antioxidants; these have a protective effect against heart disease and cancers. It should be noted that the water soluble vitamins such as vitamin C can be easily destroyed by the prolonged storage of vegetables, overcooking and keeping them warm for long periods before serving.

> **Because of the importance in the diet, the World Health Organisation recommend that we have at least 400g (just under a pound in weight) of fruit and vegetables each day.**

Frozen vegetables are picked and frozen rapidly so the vitamins and minerals are retained.

In canning, some of the water soluble vitamins are lost. In drying, most of the water soluble vitamins are lost. In making fruit juices most of the fibre is lost. Smoothies may retain a lot of the fibre.

When preparing fruit and vegetables, try to retain the vitamins by:

- preparing as late as possible;
- cooking in a minimum of water;
- keeping skins and peel on vegetables; and
- keeping vegetables warm for a minimum time.

FRUIT AND VEGETABLES

- **5 portions of fruit and vegetables may protect against chronic diseases, such as cancer and heart disease**

- **A portion of fruit or vegetables means:**
  - **Half a large fruit (e.g. avocado, grapefruit)**
  - **1 medium sized vegetable or fruit (e.g. apple, pear, banana)**
  - **2 small fruits (e.g plums)**
  - **1 cup of small fruits (e.g. grapes)**
  - **A tablespoon of dried fruits (e.g. dates)**
  - **2-3 tablespoons cooked or canned fruit**
  - **2 tablespoons cooked, frozen or canned vegetables**
  - **A bowl of salad**
  - **A glass of fruit juice (only counts as one portion each day)**

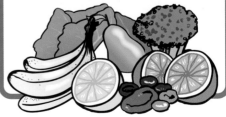

Bread, cereals, rice, pasta and potatoes ▼

These foods are the preferred source of energy for our bodies. They all provide starchy carbohydrates. Carbohydrate provides 3.75kcal per g.

As well as carbohydrates these foods provide a range of B vitamins.

Wholemeal breads, brown rice, brown pasta and wholegrain breakfast cereals all have more fibre than the white varieties, which have been more highly processed or refined.

When making white flour the millers remove much of the outer husk of the wheat grain; this husk contains the fibre. Also calcium, iron and B vitamins are lost, so these are replaced.

Such foods as fortified breakfast cereals have extra B vitamins.

QUESTION

What ways can you increase the amount of starchy carbohydrate in the diet?

ANSWER

Serve bread with meals. Use thick slices of bread in making sandwiches. Use larger portions of rice, pasta, cous cous, noodles or potatoes.

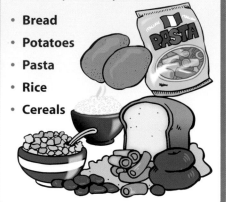

Bread, cereals, rice, pasta and potatoes

These provide energy, some protein, calcium and iron, B vitamins. Wholegrain varieties are high in fibre.

Need to encourage diet high in starchy carbohydrates.

- **Bread**
- **Potatoes**
- **Pasta**
- **Rice**
- **Cereals**

Meat, fish and alternatives ▼

These foods are important sources of protein, iron and zinc. They also provide B vitamins. Meat, fish and eggs also provide vitamin B12 but nuts and pulses do not provide this vitamin.

For anyone who is a vegetarian or vegan it is important that they take adequate iron and protein from pulses, nuts and soya products. To reduce the amount of fat taken, lean meat should be used and the skin trimmed from poultry.

Milk and dairy foods ▼

Milk and dairy products are rich in calcium, protein, B vitamins and also provide some vitamin A. Pasteurizing and sterilizing milk help to preserve it. Milk also contains vitamin B12. Some people are intolerant to milk, and are usually advised to take soya products instead. To reduce the fat in the diet use semi-skimmed or skimmed milk, low fat yoghurt and cottage cheese.

Foods containing fats and sugars ▼

These foods add variety and flavour but they are high in fat and sugar and hence calories. They can contribute to health problems such as obesity, coronary heart disease and dental disease if eaten in excess.

Often people, especially children, eat large portions of these foods, which means their diet is unbalanced.

QUESTION

What alternative snacks are there to potato crisps, sweets and chocolate?

ANSWER

Fruit, dried fruit, seeds, plain nuts, plain biscuits and vegetable sticks.

Fluids including alcohol ▼

Fluids containing caffeine and alcohol act as diuretics causing the body to excrete extra urine. Alcohol also has an adverse effect on the liver. It contributes to the development of liver cirrhosis and obesity if taken in excess.

It is recommended that people do not take excessive amounts of alcohol.

For health, women should not take more than 21 units of alcohol per week and men 28 units per week.

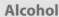

Alcohol

	Alcohol
• Beer/lager/cider	3-6%
• Wines	9-13%
• Spirits	37-45%
• Liqueurs	20-40%
• Fortified wines	18-25%

• **Absorbed in stomach**

• **Broken down in liver**

• **7 calories per gram**

• **Unit of alcohol = 8 grams**

• **Half pint of beer, lager, cider (300ml)**
• **Glass of wine (100ml)**
• **Tot of spirits (25ml)**

Nutrition and life stages ▼

Good nutrition is important throughout the whole of life. People need different amounts of energy depending on their gender, activity level and state of health.

Babies ▼

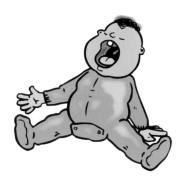

Breast milk is the ideal food for the growing infant. Babies grow rapidly during the first few months of life and breast milk provides all of the nutrients that a baby requires for health in this period. The milk provides about 700kcal per day for the infant.

If the mother is unable to breast-feed then an infant formula milk can be used. These formulae are made from cow's milk which is adapted to provide a composition as similar as possible to breast milk. These formulae must be correctly made up, as if they are over-concentrated they can put an excessive load on the babies developing kidneys.

Weaning ▼

Solid foods (which are in a smooth puréed or liquidized form), in addition to breast or infant milk are given to a baby in the process of weaning. Such foods are given from the age of 6 months.

It is recommended that the first foods given to a baby are rice, puréed potatoes or other vegetables. A spoonful is usually introduced before either breast or infant milk feeds. The puréed foods can be home-made or commercial ones.

Gradually the amounts of solids are increased and also the texture made lumpier as the child develops teeth. During the teething stage hard items such as rusks or pieces of hard vegetable such as carrots are useful for the child to chew on under supervision to ensure no choking occurs.

By the age of a year a child should be eating a varied diet. It is not recommended that ordinary cows' milk is given to infants before a year of age but infant formula milk should be continued until then.

Pre-school children ▼

A varied diet should be continued for pre-school children without the addition of foods containing high levels of sugar or salt.

Sugar and sugary drinks provided between meals has been linked with dental decay (dental caries). Sugar promotes the growth of bacteria in the mouth and these produce acids, which erode the teeth. Therefore it is beneficial for children to be given sugary sweets and snacks at the end of meals.

Children between 1-3 years are prone to iron anaemia which can be due to inadequate amounts of iron in the diet. Therefore it is important that young children are given a good source of dietary iron such as red meat and if they are vegetarian a good range of iron-containing foods such as peas, beans and lentils.

Young children may choke on items such as nuts, boiled sweets and gob-stoppers, and therefore these should not be given to pre-school children.

Full cream milk should be given to young children. Semi-skimmed milk can be introduced at 2 years of age and fully skimmed milk at 5 years.

School age children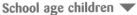

Children of this age are growing very fast and are also usually very active.

There is usually a growth spurt in children just before the onset of puberty (ages 11-13 years). It is important to offer children a varied diet with plenty of energy from large portions of starchy carbohydrates, plenty of fruits and vegetables and a good source of calcium and protein from milk and milk-containing foods.

Dental health is important and a diet with excessive frequent sugar consumption is not recommended.

Children also need a high intake of calcium due to skeletal growth. This can be provided by milk, cheese and fish with small bones.

Adolescents ▼

The nutritional needs of adolescents are high because of the growth and activity that occurs. Adolescents usually go through the end of a growth spurt with extra requirements for energy, calcium and protein.

Breakfast eating ▼

Breakfast has long been recognised as an important meal. It is vital not from just a nutritional view but the way it enhances cognitive performance and hence the ability of children to learn. Initiatives such as 'breakfast clubs' have been incorporated into some schools.

School lunches ▼

Nutritional recommendations on school meals are being introduced to make them healthier.

QUESTION

What breakfast options are there for a teenager?

ANSWER

Fruit juice, porridge, and semi-skimmed milk OR fruit juice, cereal and semi-skimmed milk and toast with spread OR fruit juice, grilled bacon sandwich OR fruit smoothie and cereal bar.

Women

Adult women need to have a well-balanced and varied diet without excessive amounts of energy and fat to prevent obesity developing. For the average women a diet providing 30% of the energy from fat would contain about 70g of fat.

Iron is important in a woman's diet to meet the needs of the body and to counteract the monthly blood loss. The iron requirements for women are greater than those of men.

Calcium is also important in a woman's diet to maintain the bone structure of the skeleton.

For any women contemplating becoming pregnant or who are pregnant a supplement of folic acid should be taken. Normally 400 micrograms of folic acid is recommended each day for the first 12 weeks of pregnancy. This helps to prevent neural tube defects such as spina bifida.

It is important during pregnancy that the mother does not 'eat for two' and gain excessive amounts of weight, which may be difficult to lose after the baby is born.

During the period of breast-feeding the mother's calorie requirements, and those for protein, calcium, phosphorus, as well as the B vitamins, vitamin C, vitamin A and D, are all increased to enable the mother to produce breast milk.

During pregnancy high levels of vitamin A can have an adverse effect on the foetus. For this reason, supplements containing vitamin A are not recommended. Also liver and foods containing it such as pâté are not recommended due to the high levels of vitamin A they contain.

Also pregnant women and the foetus are more susceptible to foodborne infections such as listeria which is found in soft cheeses made from unpasteurized milk, unwashed vegetables and chilled foods.

Men ▼

Men have a higher energy requirement than women due to them having a general higher activity level than women and also a greater muscle mass in the body.

Men require more zinc than women for sexual functioning.

Coronary heart disease is more common in men than women and therefore it is important that men avoid this by watching the amount of saturated fat in their diet, ensuring that they take plenty of fruit and vegetables and avoid becoming obese.

Many men become obese because of a lifestyle with too little exercise and too many calories, which can often be derived from fat and excess alcohol.

Elderly people ▼

Elderly people vary a great deal in their activity levels, nutritional status and health. If elderly people do not go out of doors they may not get vitamin D from sunlight. If elderly people do not eat fruit and vegetables or meat due to poor teeth they can lack in vitamins and minerals. Some elderly people find shopping and preparing food difficult.

Malnutrition ▼

The term malnutrition means unbalanced or disordered eating and results in adverse consequences to health. It is often considered in the context of underdeveloped countries and the situation of starvation. However, it can be applied to situations where too much is eaten and problems like obesity develop.

Undernutrition - too little of nutrients ▼

- **Scurvy** - lack of vitamin C.

- **Iron deficiency anaemias**
  Symptoms include:
    - tiredness;   • listlessness; and   • pale mucous membranes.

It can also delay wound healing. Tannin in tea and unprocessed bran decreases non haem iron absorption. Groups at risk are:

Elderly people

- **Many older people do not have enough vitamin D in their diet, which is necessary for bone health**

- **Some older people have low intakes of some vitamins (e.g. folate and vitamin C) and minerals**

- **Those without their own teeth, living in institutions or from lower socio-economic groups, are at the highest risk of vitamin and mineral deficiencies**

Women of child bearing age - menstrual blood loss causes loss of iron. Those with heavy periods are particularly prone; also during pregnancy and after the delivery of the baby.

Elderly people - poor diet, poor absorption. Many elderly people have a poor diet because of factors such as no teeth, not cooking meals; also, as people age, their absorption of minerals is reduced.

Toddlers - poor diet with little meat or iron containing foods.

Those who take little meat or fish.

- **Constipation and bowel cancer** - lack of fibre, NSP.
- **Starvation** - too few calories.
- **Rickets** - vitamin D and calcium - seen in children of mainly Asian origin.

Overnutrition - too many nutrients ▼
This is far more common in this country.

- **Obesity** - due to too many calories being taken and stored as fat.
- **Coronary heart disease** - related to excess saturated fat and other factors such as obesity.
- **High blood pressure** - related to obesity and excess salt.
- **Dental decay** - related to too much sugar taken too frequently, especially between meals, and poor dental hygiene.

Obesity can result in other problems.

Problems associated with obesity

- **Heart disease**
- **Hypertension**
- **Joint problems**
- **Breathlessness**
- **Type 2 diabetes**
- **Strokes**
- **Varicose veins**
- **Accidents**
- **Certain cancers**
- **Poor recovery from surgery**
- **Psychological problems**
- **Social problems**

QUESTION

What 3 things can you do to improve the diet of those you care for?

ANSWER

Advise them to: 1. Include plenty of fruit and vegetables in their diet. 2. Drink between 6-8 cups (2 litres (3 pints) of water a day 3. Eat less fatty and sugary foods.

Summary ▼

As can be seen, malnutrition is prevalent in the UK with obesity, coronary heart disease, cancers as well as different types of anaemia being common. Think what you can do to help prevent this for yourself, in your own family and with those you care for.

'Eating healthily is all about balancing the diet'

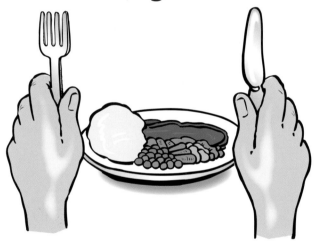

Appendix 1 ▼
Glossary ▼

FSA - Food Standards Agency
The Food Standards Agency provide information on nutrition and diet.

The Balance of Good Health
A pictorial model of a healthy diet, the model comprises a plate with 5 segments showing each type of foods required for a healthy balanced diet.

NSP - Non-starch polysaccharide
An alternate name for dietary fibre.

DRV - Dietary Reference Value
The term used to cover LRNI, EAR, RNI and safe intake. See Department of Health, report on Health and Social Subjects: 41. Dietary Reference Values for Food Energy and Nutrients for the United Kingdom, HMSO (London, 1991).

EAR - Estimated Average Requirement
The estimated average requirement of a group of people for energy or protein or a vitamin or mineral. About half will usually need more than the EAR, and half less.

RNI - Reference Nutrient Intake
The reference nutrient intake for protein or a vitamin or a mineral. An amount of the nutrient that is enough, or more than enough, for about 97% of the people in the group. If average intake of a group is at the RNI, then the risk of deficiency in the group is small.

Gram
A unit of weight, approximately 6 grams to a teaspoon.

Obesity
Excessive deposition of body fat.

BMR - Basal Metabolic Rate
The rate the body uses energy for keeping us alive.

Amino acids
Small components of proteins.

Fatty acids
Acids found in fats.

Intrinsic sugars
Any sugar which is contained within the cell wall of a food.

Extrinsic sugars
Any sugar which is not contained within cell walls of food. Examples are sugars in honey, table sugar and lactose in milk and milk products.

Electrolytes
Sodium and potassium which are responsible for fluid balance.

Appendix 2 ▼

Example test questions ▼

1. **How many sections are there in the Balance of Good Health?**

2. **What does DRV stand for?**

3. **What foods do many people eat too little of?**

4. **What is the vitamin made by the action of sunlight on the skin?**

5. **How many portions of fruit and vegetables should we eat each day?**

6. **How much fluid should a person drink each day?**

7. **What does BMR stand for?**

8. **The deficiency associated with lack of iron is?**

9. **What is high blood pressure related to?**

10. **What should people with diabetes avoid in large amounts?**

ANSWERS

Question 1: 5	Question 6: 2 litres or 3 pints
Question 2: Dietary Reference Value	Question 7: Basal Metabolic Rate
Question 3: Fruit and vegetables	Question 8: Iron deficiency anaemia
Question 4: Vitamin D	Question 9: Salt and obesity
Question 5: 5	Question 10: Sugar